Flourishing Fatima

Playing with switch scanning

Created by Luke Thompson

Co-author Caroline Bennett

Illustrated by Kat Willott

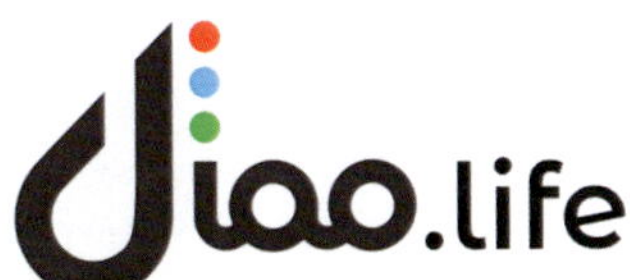

Published by Jiao Ltd

Jiao.life

Scan the QR codes to access the digital book or listen to the audio book.

Audiobook

Digital Book

The Seven Stages of Switch Development

Flourishing Fatima is part of the Switch Heroes, social stories created to support switch-users with their Switch progression. The Switch Heroes series is part of the Seven Stages of Switch Development, created by Occupational Therapist and AT specialist Luke Thompson.

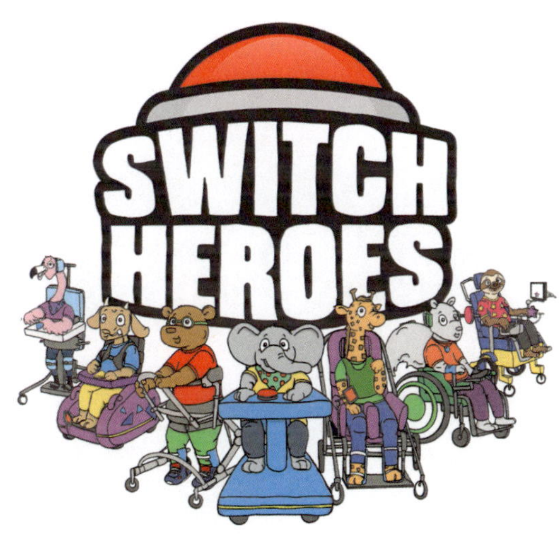

Fatima loves her stories

Do you like yours too?

Now she's got her
Blue Kite switch

Fatima can choose!

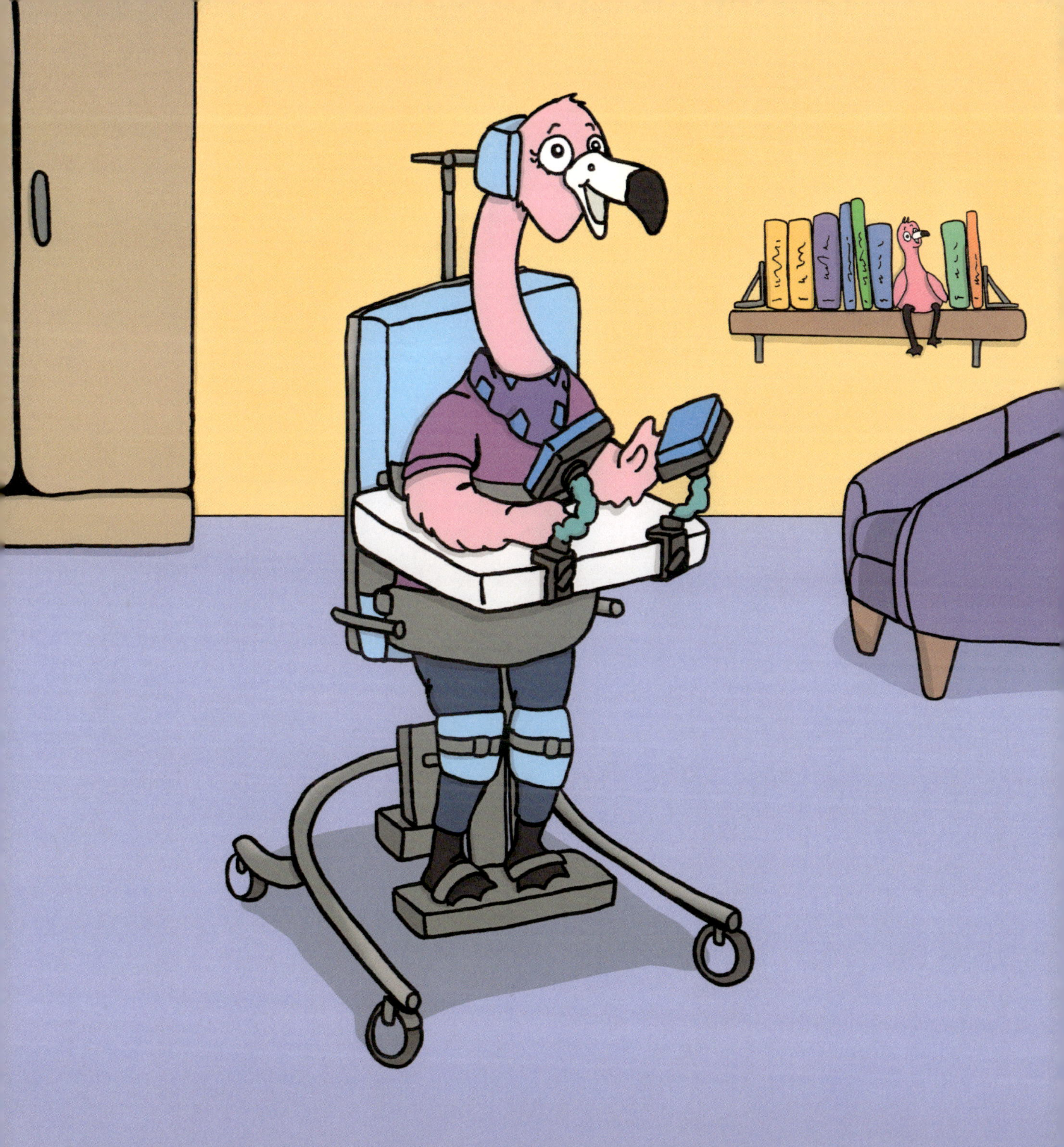

Can you see her switch?

It's plugged into this box

So Fatima can choose her book

About a chick, a plane or fox

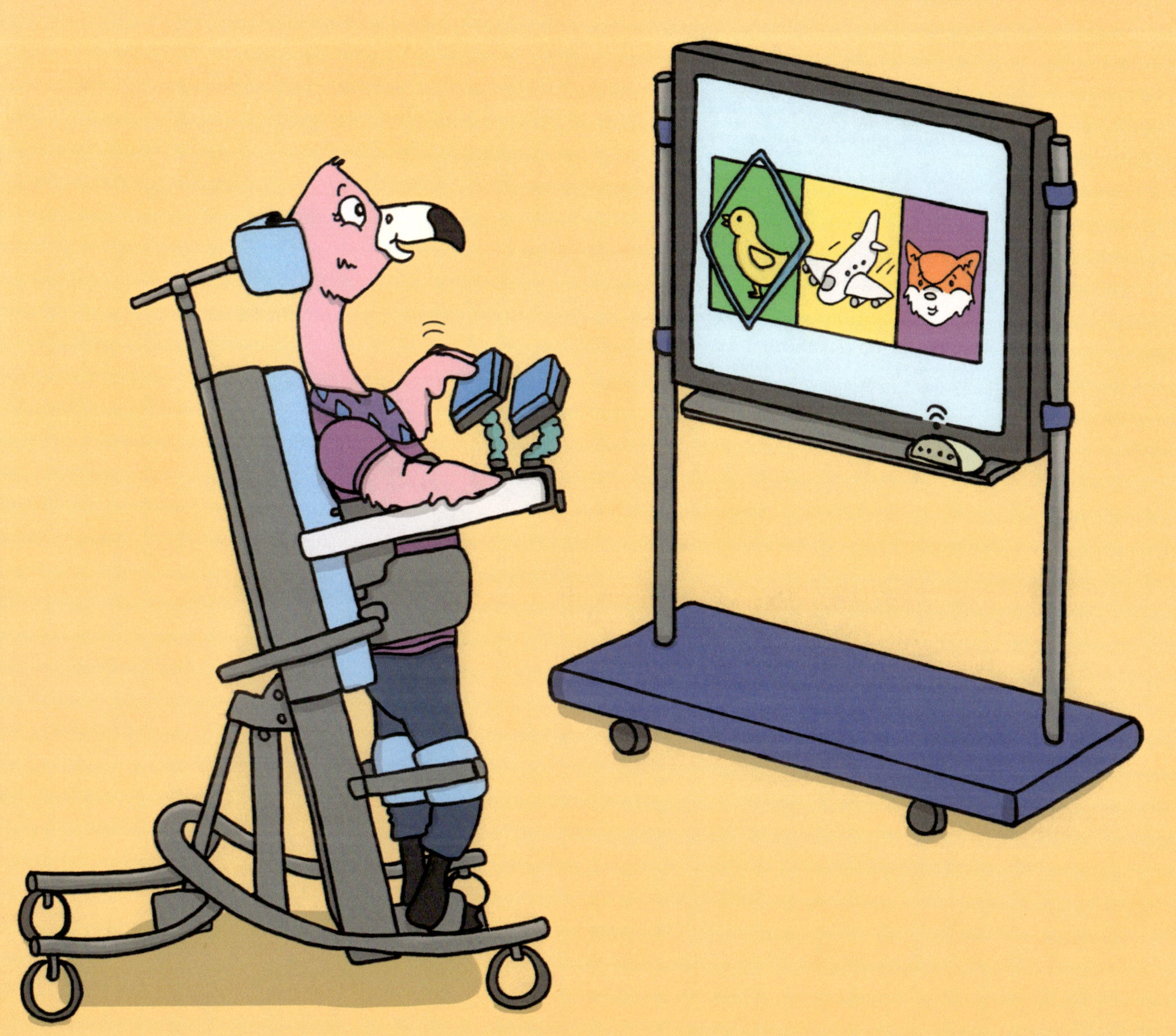

Would you like a try?

This box is an interface

Plug in your switch, scan, select

A book on football,
dance, or space

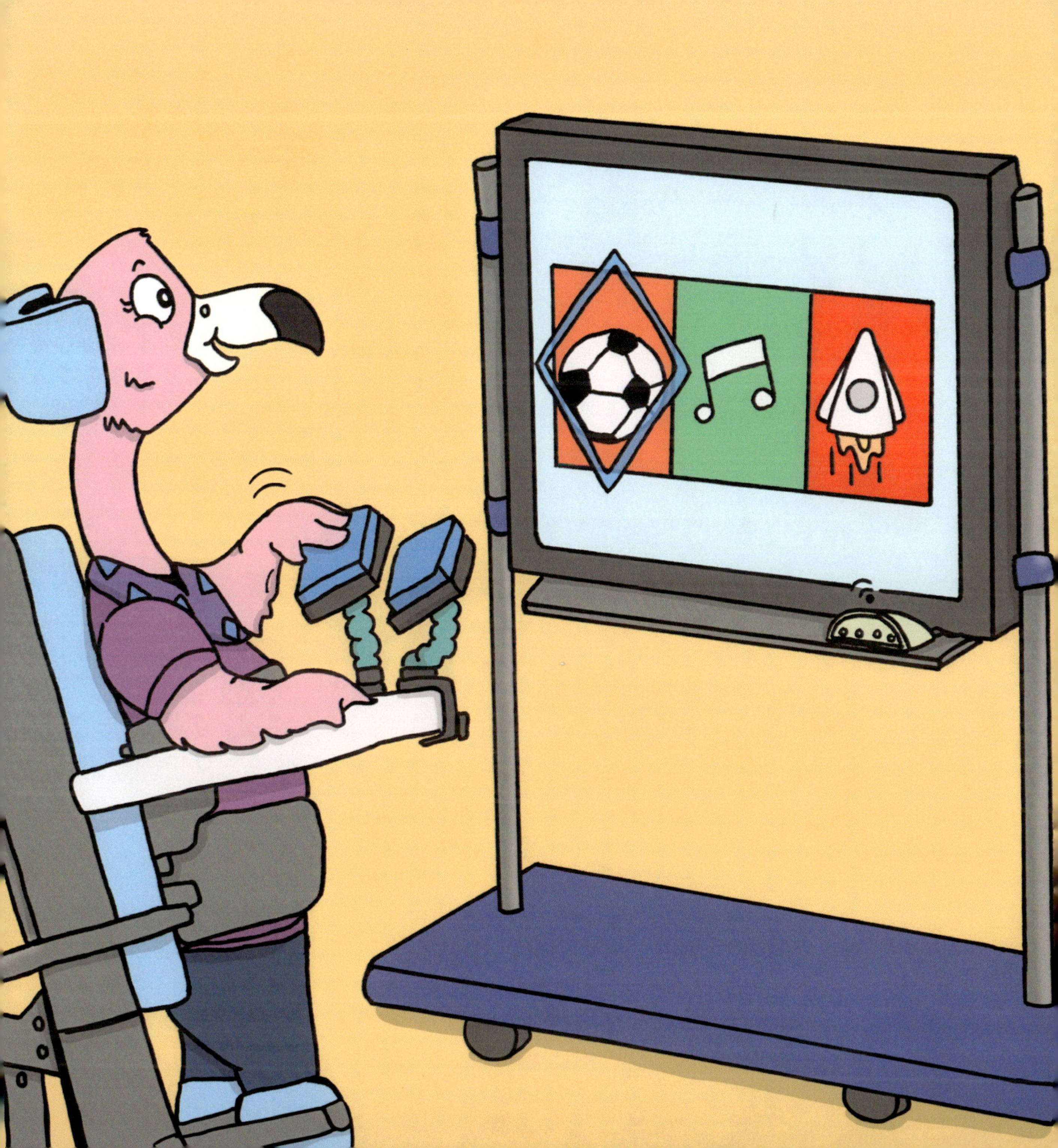

Every time you push the switch

The options move along

Then you press the other switch

To pick your chosen one

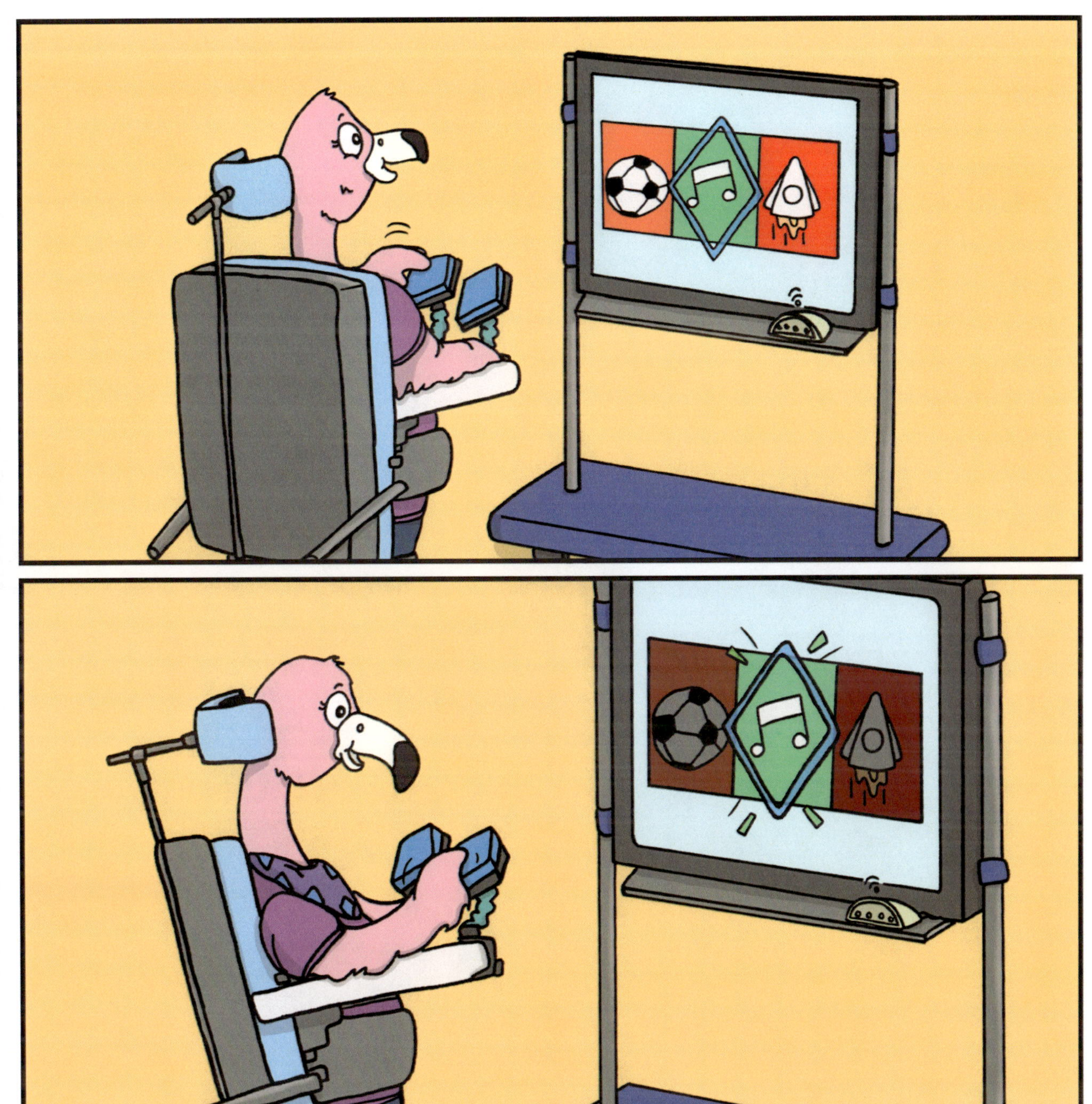

You really are quite clever

Making choices with your switch

Fatima, thanks for showing us

We'll use this quite a bit

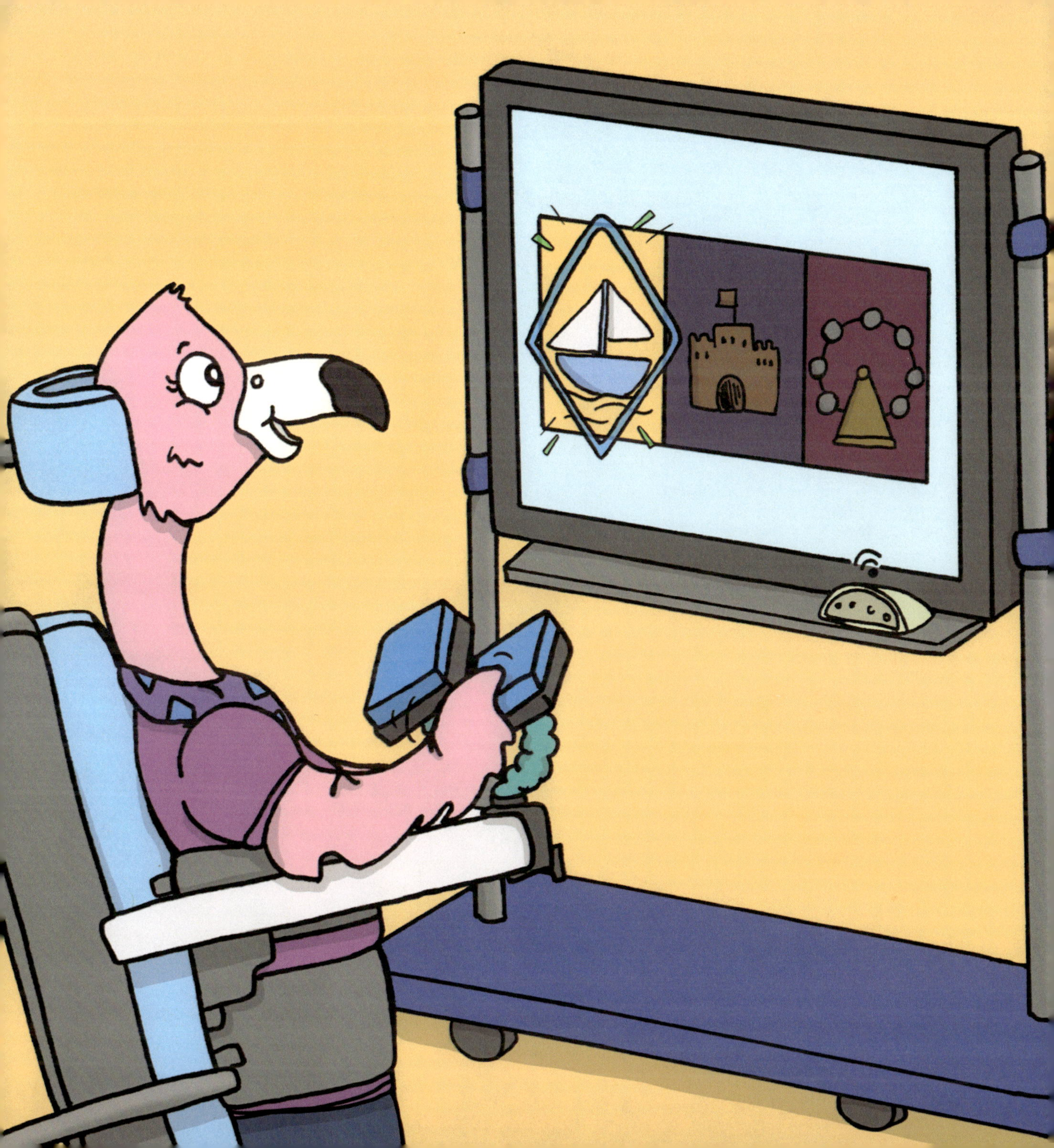

Isn't it quite brilliant
These big switch interfaces?

With two switches
and marvellous skills

You're going places

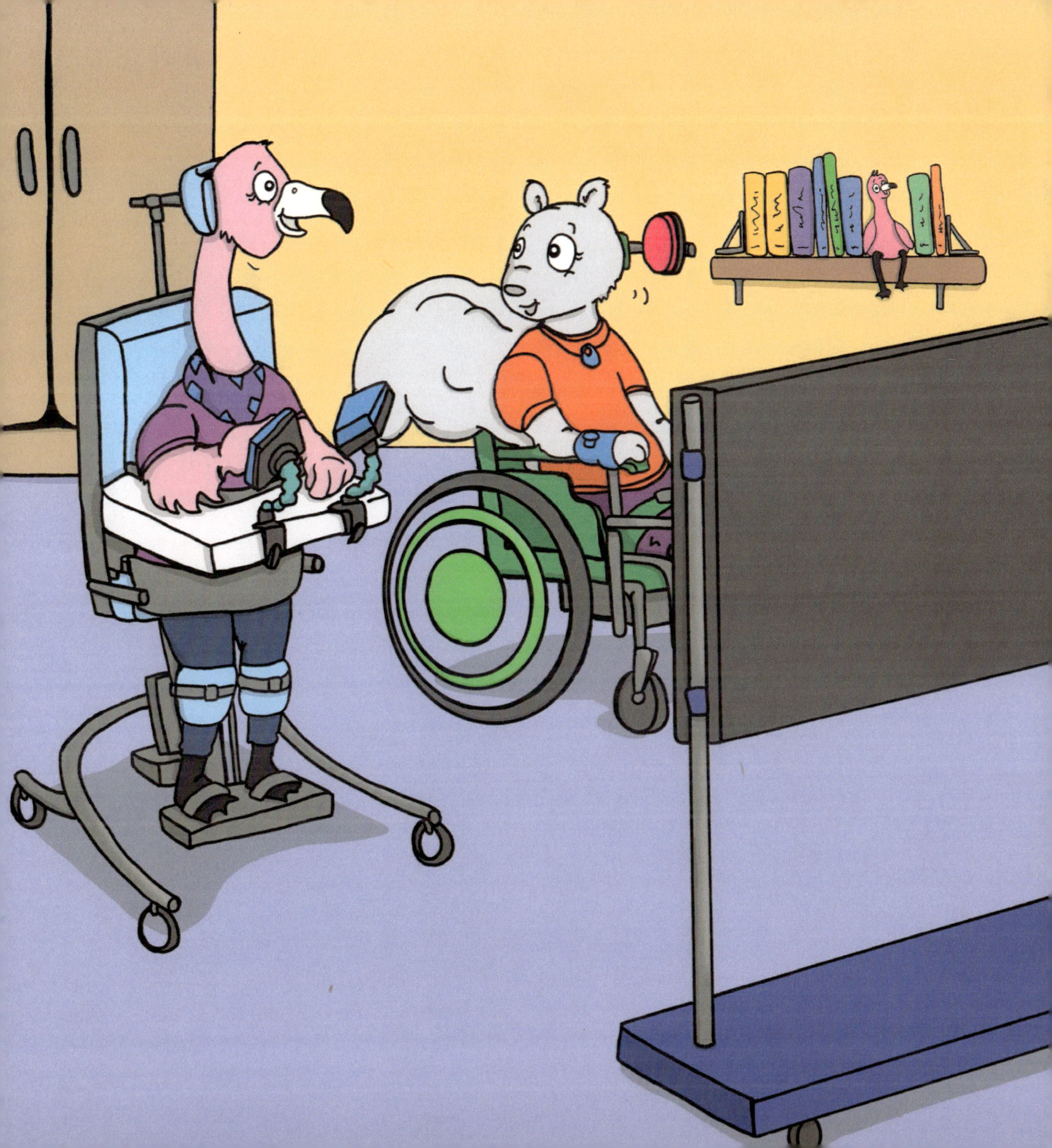

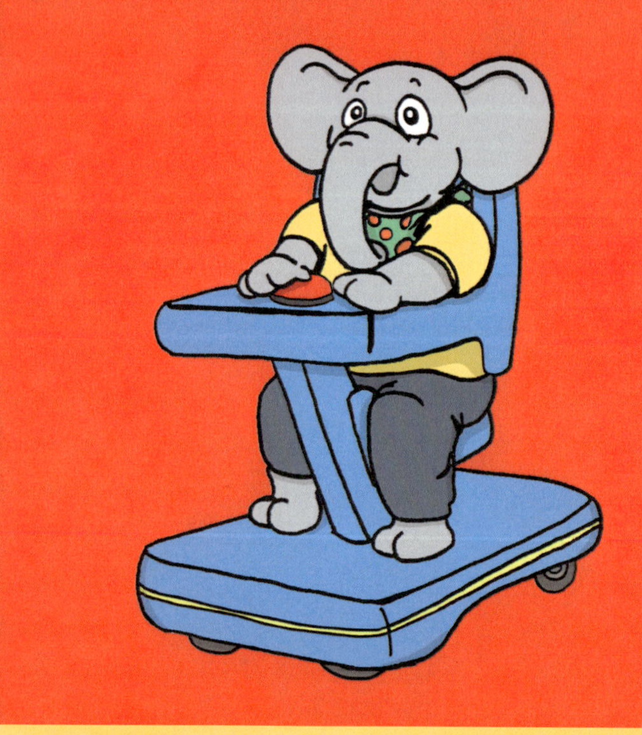
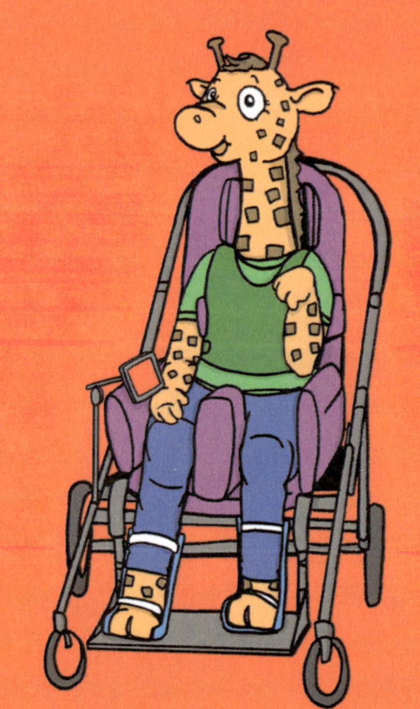
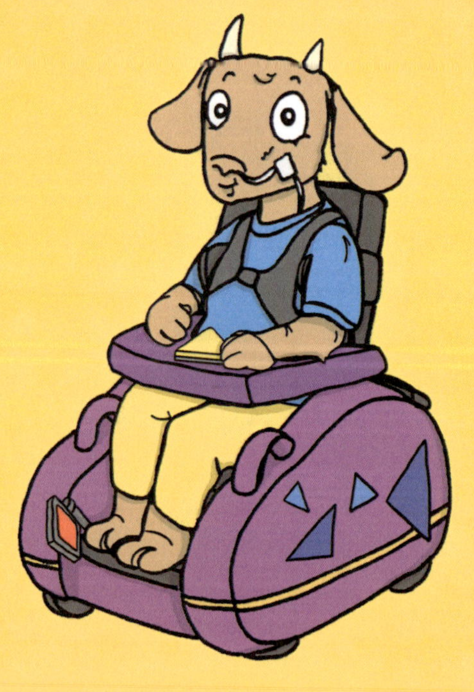
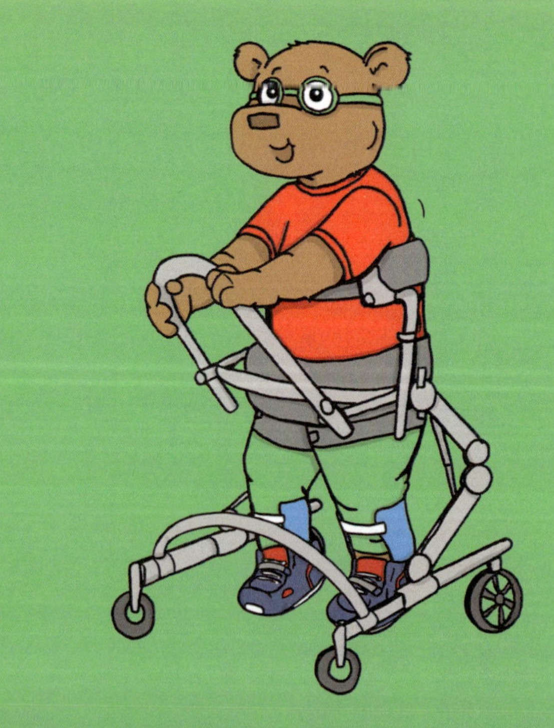

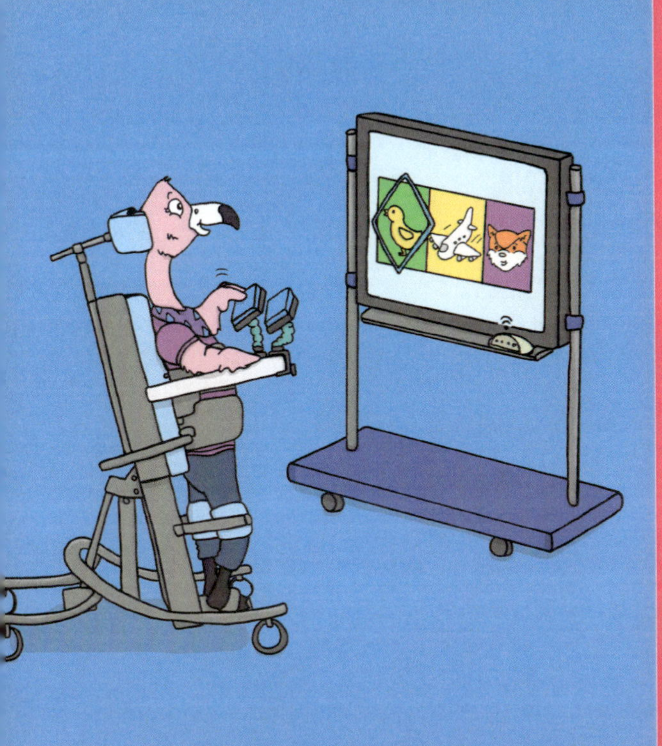

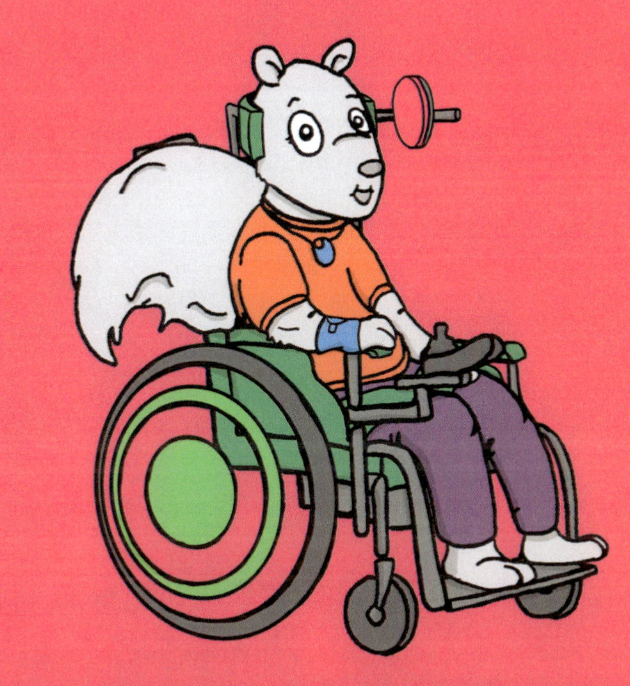

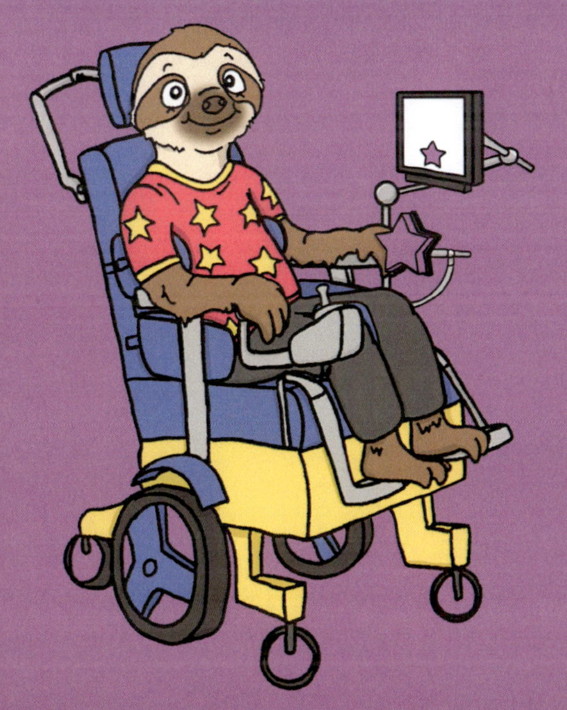

Photo of you!

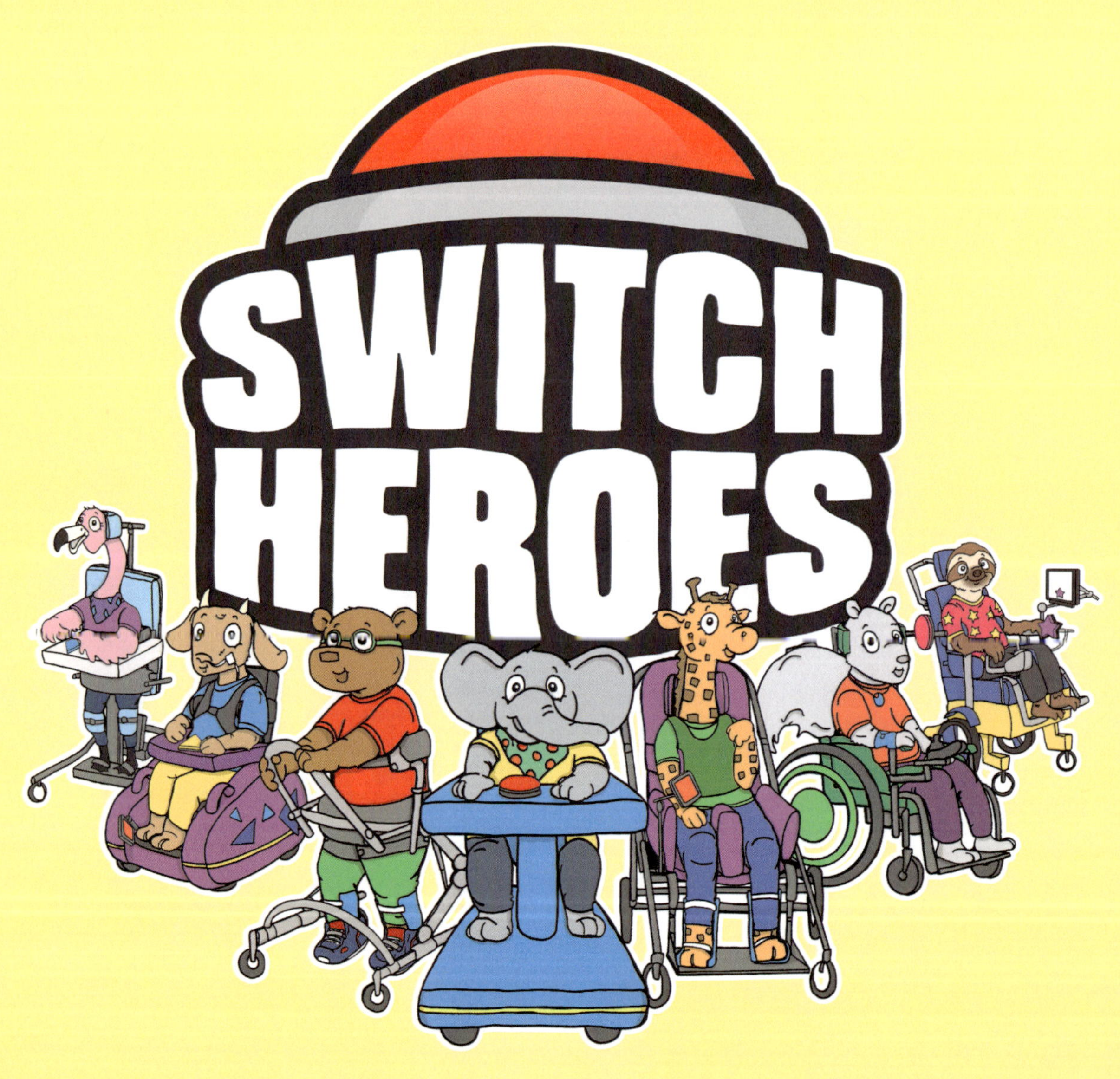
SWITCH
HEROES

The Seven Stages of Switch Development

The Seven Stages of Switch Development is a resource designed for switch-users, their families, caregivers and those who assist them in using switches. It features child-friendly characters and stories that support everyones learning.

The framework provides a helpful reference for measuring and tracking progress while offering flexibility to accommodate the unique needs and preferences of each switch-user.

Written directly to the switch-user, the framework can be read to them if they are unable to read it themselves. Our aim is to ensure that those supporting the child/switch-user can prioritise the child's needs and perspective in the process of developing their switch skills. We have seen the impact of involving the child in the learning process. Seeking their input and feedback regularly empowers them to take an active role in their development and combat learned helplessness.

Adapted from: Bean, I. (2011). Switch Progression Learning Journeys Road Map. Inclusive Technology. Burkhart, L. (2018). Stepping Stones to Switch Access. Perspectives of the ASHA Special Interest Groups, 3(12), pp.33-44. doi:https://doi/10.1044/persp3.sig12.33.

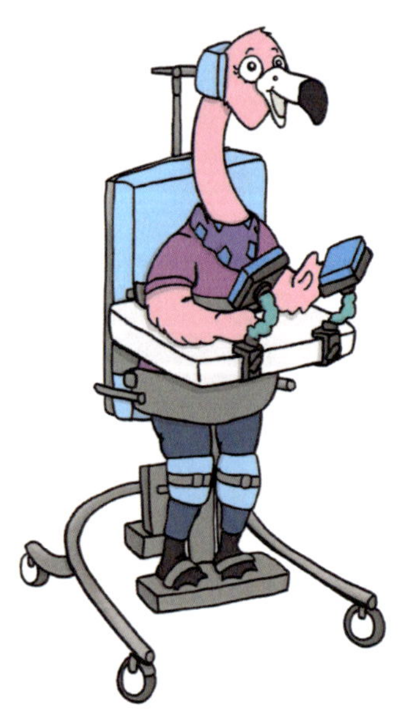

Definition

Flourishing Fatima is the stage where you are introduced to the concept of switch-scanning. This is where you use two switches to scan and select or get. The 'scan' switch moves through options by repeated presses and the 'select' or 'get' switch is pressed to activate or confirm a choice. Here you are more explicitly learning about choice. Choice will now progressively grow as you develop through this stage.

Switch-scanning activities at this stage are very simple, error-friendly learning. This means activities are really easy to make a choice but there is little pressure on the outcome of the choice. 'Oops' are the best way we learn, and it is helpful for someone to give us feedback if they notice. For example, Oops I think you wanted to choose the apple, but you choose the banana instead and you looked unhappy/frustrated?

You can use one switch with timed options (automatically scans the options, switch is set to start scan and then select/get) but this is a lot trickier than using two.

Playing with switch-scanning: You've started to master switch-scanning, understand it well and using it confidently. You can move through options using the 'scan' switch and confirm your choices independently with the 'select/get' switch

You're becoming very independent in your decision-making! You can choose from a increasing range of options on your own and showing preferences in your choice (rather than just making random selections)

You are familiar with playing/using a range of switch-scanning games and activities

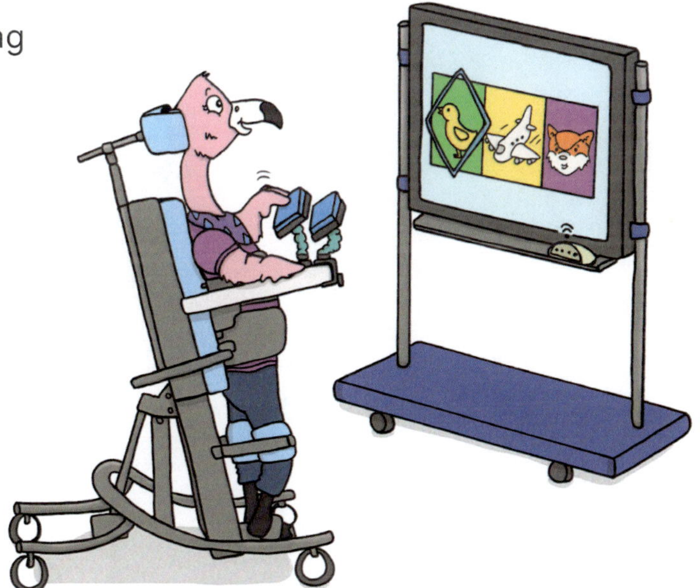

- You don't have to use specialist software; you can manually teach scanning with two audio output switches (or one with two-switch option) with 'move' and 'get' recorded on them. Then you can use a finger or a cut out frame to become the scan box

- Start with two options and slowly add more choices as the child develops

- Do not attempt to influence the switch-user to the choice they should make

- Use the phrase 'something different' if the child seems frustrated with the options

- Introduce the scanning method in a clear and structured way

- Use activities and materials that are motivating and engaging for the user

- Provide clear and consistent feedback to reinforce successful scanning and switch activations

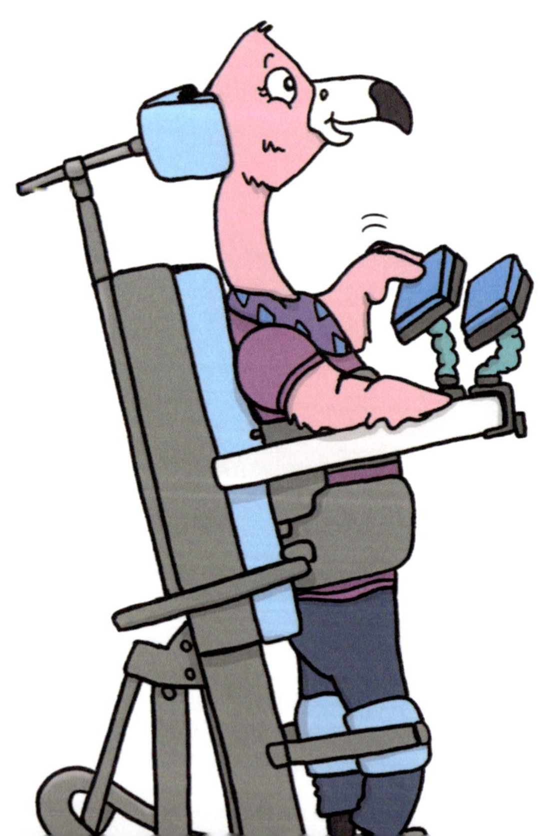

Activities

- Use software designed for creating nursery rhymes to write your own by selecting characters, story lines, and other aspects of the story through multiple choices at each step

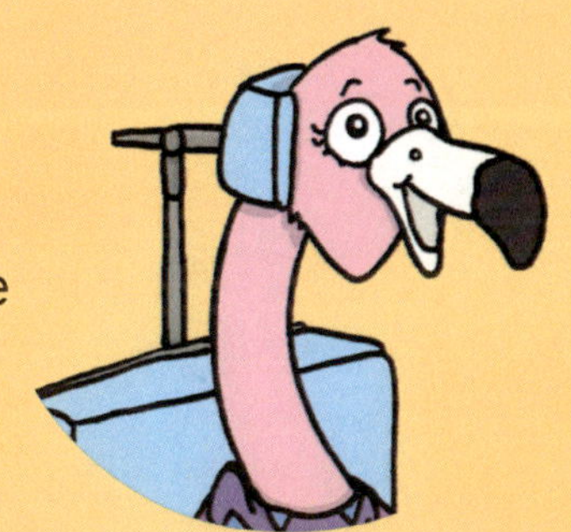

- Set up a page in a high-tech, grid-based communication aid that enables the child to scan and select activities. Start with a small number of options and gradually increase them as the child's skills and abilities develop

- Write a story using two switches. Use a voice-output switch programmed with a list of motivating options such as animals, colours, people etc. Then programme another switch to say, 'that's it!'

Instead of a prompt hierarchy where the type of prompt increase in support level, we recommend our one prompt switch support cycle. Find out more at Jiao.life

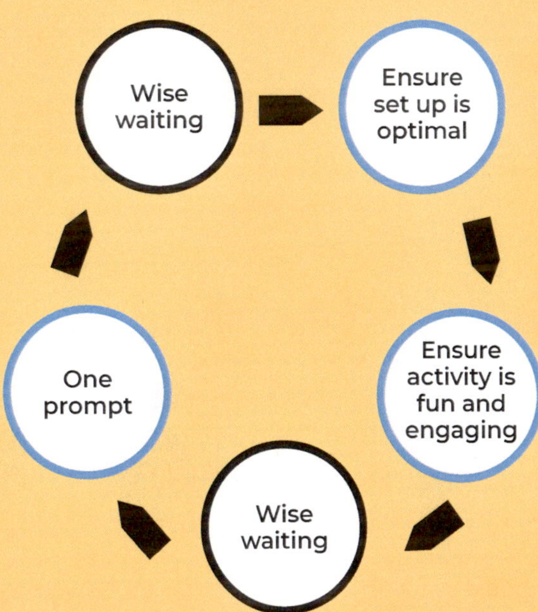

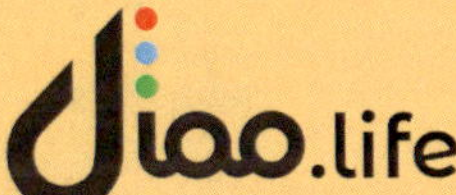

The Assessment Tool

Proficient step							
Consolidating step							
Emerging step							
Emerging – Developing – Consolidating – Proficient (cognitive, physical skill required for each stage)							
Physical	E D C P	E D C P	E D C P	E D C P	E D C P	E D C P	E D C P
Cognitive	E D C P	E D C P	E D C P	E D C P	E D C P	E D C P	E D C P

The Seven Stages of Switch Development ▶

Stage 1 Exploring Egbert	Stage 2 Journeying Jiao	Stage 3 Growing Gareth	Stage 4 Budding Brayton	Stage 5 Flourishing Fatima	Stage 6 Succeeding Saffi	Stage 7 Celebrating Syed
Learning by experience – single switch	Making something happen – single switch	Playing with two switches Making two things happen	Two switches one activity	Switch scanning – failure Free	Switch scanning – finding the right one	Independent in functional switch use

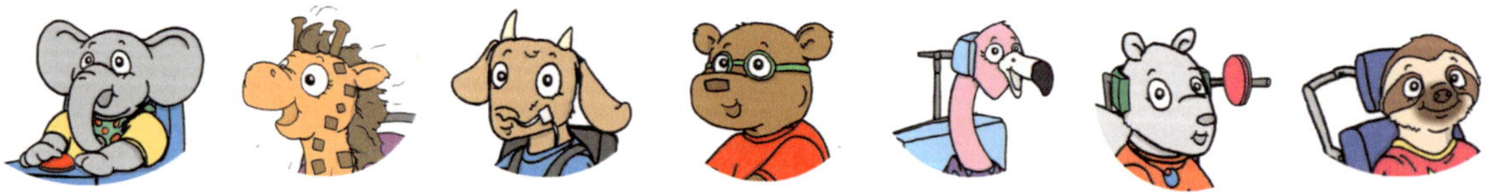

Print version available at **Jiao.life**

How to use the assessment tool

- The stages of switch development are not mutually exclusive, so progress can be made across multiple stages simultaneously

- Once a step is completed, mark it off and add the date

- The assessment tool can be used for goal setting, where helpers can add target dates and change the text/box colour accordingly

- There is a stream for assessing cognitive and physical skill development, divided into four steps for each stage (Emerging, Developing, Consolidating and Proficient)

- Helpers should consider the cognitive and physical skills required for each level

- This additional stream can help identify areas that may require additional support and highlight strengths and weaknesses for targeted interventions

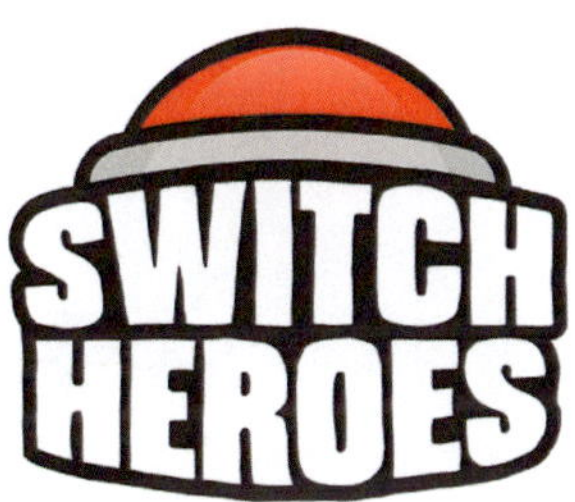

At Jiao Ltd, we are dedicated to empowering individuals through innovative assistive technology solutions.

We provide personalised services and training to help children, families, and professionals navigate the world of assistive tech. For more resources, training options, or to learn how we can support you, visit Jiao.life or get in touch with us directly. We look forward to hearlng from you!

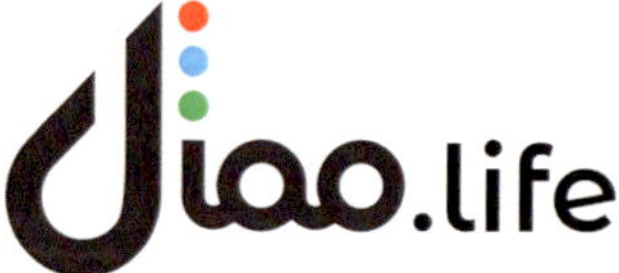

This is to certify that

____

is playing with
switch scanning

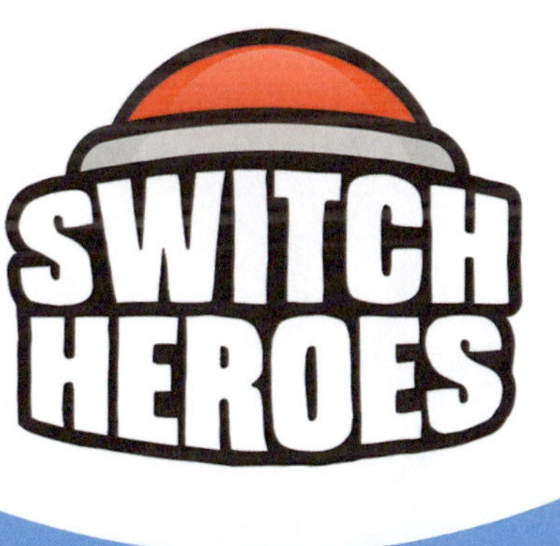

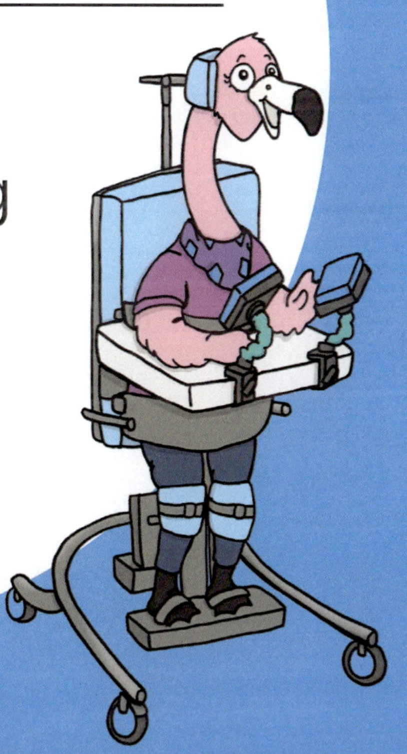

Notes

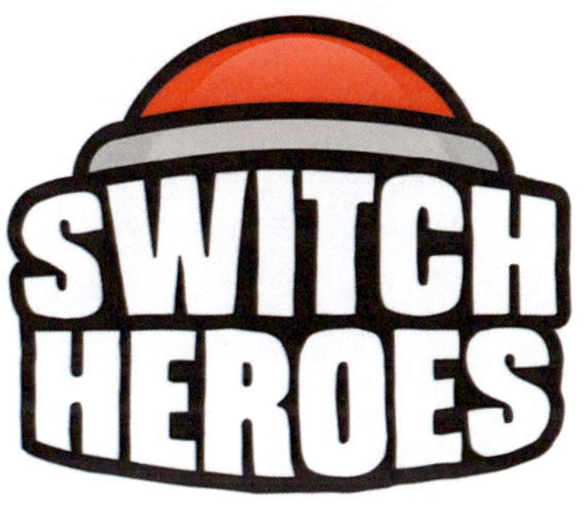